Gut Health and Longevity

How to Heal Your Gut, Restore Your Health, and Live a Longer, Happier Life

Carl B. Mariscal

Table of content

Introduction...3

Chapter 1: Understanding the Gut-Health Connection...................................6

    1.1 Introduction to Gut Health...................6

    1.2 How Gut Health Impacts Overall Well-being...... 9

    1.3 Common Gut Health Issues.............17

Chapter 2: Building a Foundation for Gut Health.... 27

    2.1 The Role of Nutrition in Gut Health..................27

    2.2 Hydration and Its Impact on Digestion.............34

    2.3 Balancing Gut Health with Lifestyle Choices... 38

Chapter 3: A Healthy Gut Diet.................... 43

    3.1 Foods to Avoid for Optimal Gut Health............. 43

    3.2 Meal Ideas for a healthy gut........................... 46

Chapter 4: Lifestyle Practices for a Healthy Gut..... 51

    4.1 Stress Management and Gut Health................ 51

    4.2 Exercise and Its Impact on Digestion............... 59

    4.3 Sleep, Circadian Rhythms, and Gut Health...... 63

    4.4 The Gut-Brain Connection.............................. 69

    4.5 Holistic Approaches to Gut Health.................... 76

Chapter 5:Working with Healthcare Professionals. 81

Conclusion... 90

Introduction

Among our everyday struggles and goals, among the busy symphony of life, we often forget about the amazing adventure occurring within our own bodies—the voyage of gut health. Trillions of microbes inhabit the human gut, a fascinating and complex ecology that is essential to our general health. Greetings from the pages of this book, where we will set off on an amazing journey into the core of your well-being.

Gut health is more than just a catchphrase; it is a profound realisation that our mental and physical well-being is intricately linked to the vibrant microcosm that lives within our digestive systems. We will explore the amazing intricacy of the gut and learn how it impacts not just our digestion but also our immune system, mental health, and other areas as we unravel the secrets of the stomach in these chapters.

We're going to take you on a tour through the nutrition labyrinth, illuminating the power of foods that nourish your gut microbes and yourself. You'll discover the wonders of fiber, the advantages of probiotics and prebiotics, and how kitchen decisions can change your life.

However, it goes beyond what's on your plate. This book serves as your compass in the comprehensive undertaking that is gut health. We'll explore how your lifestyle choices might affect the balance of your digestive system. We'll look at how every element of your life may affect your gut, from stress management to the benefits of consistent exercise and restorative sleep.

That is not where the trip ends. We'll explore the mind-gut connection, an intriguing conversation that occurs between your stomach and brain and has a significant impact on your mental and emotional health. This relationship clarifies how our emotions and ideas may influence our digestive health and vice versa.

Lastly, we'll provide you with the know-how to diagnose and treat gut health problems and advise you on when and how to work with medical experts. We are here to provide you with the information and understanding you need to confidently navigate your route to a healthy gut and a more fulfilled life.

Chapter 1: Understanding the Gut-Health Connection

1.1 Introduction to Gut Health

In a nutshell, gut health is good health. Since your gastrointestinal tract is part of your gut, "gut health" describes the general state of that system, including the bacteria that live there. Adhere to us!

After food is transported from your mouth to your stomach, your GI absorbs the nutrients and energy it contains and excretes the remaining material. That in and of itself is a very significant task, but research has shown that our stomachs are responsible for much more than just digesting the avocado toast you had for the morning. We now know that our intestines influence a wide range of other elements of our health, including immunity, chronic disease, and brain function.

Although it may not seem very glamorous, 70% of our immune system is located in our stomach. It is crucial to maintain good gut health to feel well since this is the area where we produce nutrients, process hormones, and detoxifying enzymes, neutralize infections, and create neurotransmitters."

Furthermore, for your stomach to function properly, it needs an army of bacteria, fungi, and other microbes. Fun fact: about 39 million microbial cells compared to 30 million human cells means that the microorganisms in and on your body may outweigh your human cells (though this is debatable). Even though these little cells only account for 3% of our body weight, they have a significantly greater impact on our general health than the actual area they occupy on and inside our bodies. We'll go into more detail on the microbiome—a system of bacteria and other microorganisms—in the next post. Additionally, there are healthy and nasty microorganisms in your stomach, just like in any community.

Not only do your gut bacteria aid in food digestion, but they also support your body's general homeostasis. Research is only starting to uncover a connection between sickness and the bacteria in your gut. Although the exact relationship is still unknown, it is most likely symbiotic—the disease is caused by harmful bacteria in the gut, and vice versa. Maintaining a balance between the "good" and "bad" bacteria that are present in all of us is essential for gut health. For instance, the stomach is home to both microorganisms that cause and combat inflammation. We are aware that we need both (consider swelling after an accident vs persistent joint inflammation). However, if this equilibrium is upset, it may create the conditions for illness to spread. Reduced immunological function, an increased risk of allergies, diabetes, multiple sclerosis, and several malignancies have all been related to specific gut bacteria. Studies have shown a connection to neurological conditions including dementia, depression, and anxiety. People with varied body proportions tend to have variable gut health, which suggests that gut health and susceptibility to obesity may be related.

1.2 How Gut Health Impacts Overall Well-being

For millions of years, humans have evolved to coexist alongside microorganisms.

Microbes have evolved to serve a variety of crucial functions in the human body over this period. It would be quite difficult to exist without the gut microbiota.

Your body is impacted by your gut microbiota from the time of your birth.

The first time you come into contact with bacteria is when you go through your mother's birth canal. On the other hand, fresh data indicates that infants could be exposed to some microorganisms while still in the womb.

As an individual grows, their gut microbiome diversifies, resulting in a greater variety of bacteria species being present. More variety in your microbiome is thought to be beneficial to your health.

It's interesting to note that your gut flora's variety is influenced by what you consume.

Your body is impacted by the growth of your microbiome in many ways, such as:

Breast milk digestion: Bifidobacteria are a kind of bacteria that first proliferate in the intestines of newborns. They process the growth-promoting, healthful carbohydrates found in breast milk.

Fiber digestion: Short-chain fatty acids, which are critical for gut health, are produced by certain bacteria during the fiber digestion process. Fiber may reduce the risk of cancer, heart disease, diabetes, and weight gain.

Immune system regulation: The gut microbiota has an impact on how well your immune system functions. Your body's response to infection may be regulated by the gut microbiota via interactions with immune cells.

Supporting the regulation of brain health:
Recent studies indicate that the central nervous system, which regulates brain activity, may be impacted by the gut microbiota.

As a result, the gut microbiota may impact vital body processes and have a variety of other effects on your health.

Your Weight May Be Affected by Your Gut Microbiota
Your intestines are home to hundreds of different kinds of bacteria, the majority of which are good for your health.

However, illness may result from an excess of harmful bacteria.

Gut dysbiosis, a term used to describe an imbalance between beneficial and harmful bacteria, may be linked to weight gain.

Numerous well-known studies have shown that identical twins, one of whom had obesity and the other did not, had radically different gut microbiomes. This proved that variations in the microbiome were not caused by genetics.

It's interesting to note that in one research, mice who got the microbiome of the obese twin gained more weight than mice that received the microbiome of the other twin, even though both groups had the same diet.

These findings suggest that dysbiosis of the microbiota may contribute to weight gain.

Thankfully, probiotics support a balanced microbiota and may aid with weight reduction. However, research indicates that probiotics likely have little impact on weight reduction, with most users shedding less than 2.2 pounds (1 kg).

It Impacts Digestive Health:

Irritable bowel syndrome (IBS) and inflammatory bowel disease (IBD) are two intestinal disorders that may be influenced by the microbiome.

Gut dysbiosis may be the cause of the bloating, cramps, and stomach discomfort that IBS sufferers experience. This is because the bacteria create a lot of gas and other substances that aggravate the symptoms of intestinal distress.

However, the microbiome's beneficial microorganisms may also enhance intestinal health.

Probiotics and yogurt include specific Lactobacilli and Bifidobacteria that may help close gaps between intestinal cells and stop leaky gut syndrome.

Additionally, certain species can stop disease-causing bacteria from adhering to the gut wall.

Taking specific probiotics including lactobacilli and Bifidobacteria helps lessen IBS symptoms.

It Could Impact Mental Health:
In certain respects, the gut microbiota may even be advantageous to brain health.

First, the brain produces chemicals known as neurotransmitters with the assistance of certain bacterial species. For instance, the stomach produces the majority of the antidepressant chemical serotonin.

Second, millions of nerves physically link the brain to the stomach.

Thus, by assisting in the regulation of the signals sent to the brain via these neurons, the gut microbiota may also have an impact on brain health.

Numerous studies have shown that the types of bacteria present in the intestines of individuals with different psychiatric problems vary from those of healthy individuals. This implies that brain health may be impacted by the gut microbiota.

It's unclear, however, whether this is just the result of various food and lifestyle choices.

Additionally, a limited number of studies have shown that certain probiotics help lessen the signs and symptoms of depression and other mental illnesses.

It Could Assist in Blood Sugar Regulation and Reduce the Risk of Diabetes:
Additionally, blood sugar regulation may be aided by the gut flora, which may impact the risk of type 1 and type 2 diabetes.

A new research looked at 33 babies who were at a high genetic risk of having type 1 diabetes.

It was discovered that before the beginning of type 1 diabetes, the microbiome's diversity abruptly decreased. Additionally, it was shown that a variety of harmful bacterial species were more prevalent just before type 1 diabetes started.

According to another research, blood sugar levels could differ significantly even amongst individuals who had the identical items. The kinds of bacteria in their stomachs might be the cause of this.

Heart Health May Benefit from the Gut Microbiome
Surprisingly, heart health may even be impacted by the gut microbiota.

A new research involving 1,500 participants discovered that the gut flora was crucial in boosting triglycerides and "good" HDL cholesterol.

By generating trimethylamine N-oxide, certain pathogenic species in the gut microbiome may also aggravate heart disease (TMAO).

A molecule called TMAO is involved in clogged arteries, which may result in heart attacks or strokes.

Choline and L-carnitine, which are substances present in red meat and other animal-based dietary sources, are converted to TMAO by certain bacteria within the microbiome, which may raise heart disease risk factors.

But when taken as a probiotic, other bacteria in the gut microbiome, including Lactobacilli, may help lower cholesterol.

1.3 Common Gut Health Issues

Gastroenterologists are medical professionals with a focus on digestive disorders. Proctologists, often known as colorectal surgeons, are surgeons who specialize in gastrointestinal disorders. Among the ailments they address most often are:

bloating:
Constipation is a functional condition characterised by difficulty passing stools, infrequency (less than three times per week), or incompleteness of faeces. A change in your typical routine or diet, or insufficient "roughage" or fiber in your diet, are common causes of constipation.

You struggle when you have a bowel movement when you are constipated. Small, firm stools and anal issues like haemorrhoids or fissures may result from it. Seldom is constipation an indication of a more severe medical problem.

Constipation may be managed at home by:

*Increasing your dietary intake of water and fiber.

*regular activity, with the intensity of your workouts, increased as tolerated.

*When the need strikes, move your bowels (resisting the desire produces constipation).

*Laxatives are a beneficial tool if these treatment options are unsuccessful. Always heed the directions on your laxative medication and the counsel of your medical professional.

Irritable bowel syndrome:
The functional disorder known as irritable bowel syndrome (IBS), often referred to as spastic colon,

irritable colon, or anxious stomach, causes your intestinal muscles to spasm more or less frequently than "normal." Medications, certain meals, and psychological stress are a few things that might cause IBS.

IBS symptoms include:

- cramping and soreness in the abdomen
- surplus gas
- ballooning
- alteration in bowel patterns, such as more frequent, firmer, or looser faeces than usual
- both diarrhoea and/or constipation

IBS may be managed at home by:

1. limiting your caffeine intake.
2. Increasing your intake of fiber.
3. Keep an eye out for (and avoid) the foods that give you IBS.
4. reducing stress or discovering new coping mechanisms.

5. following your doctor's prescription for medications.
6. keeping yourself well-hydrated throughout the day to prevent dehydration.
7. obtaining restful, quality sleep.

Your anal canal has dilated veins that are haemorrhoids. It's a structural illness. They are brought on by pregnancy, chronically high pressure from straining during a bowel movement, or prolonged diarrhoea. Haemorrhoids come in two varieties: internal and external.

Blood vessels on the inside of your anal entrance are called internal haemorrhoids. They get inflamed and begin to bleed as they stretch and fall into the anus. Internal haemorrhoids eventually have the potential to prolapse—that is, sink or stick—out of the anus.

Among the treatments are:

1.Changing your bowel habits to include not straining during your bowel movements, preventing constipation, and moving your bowels when you feel like it.

2.Your physician will close the vessels using ligating bands.

3.Your medical professional will surgically remove them. Only a tiny percentage of patients with really big, excruciating, and chronic haemorrhoids need surgery.

Veins on the exterior of the anus that is barely under the skin are known as external haemorrhoids. The external hemorrhoidal veins may sometimes break after straining, forming blood clots under the skin. This very painful state is referred to as a "pile."

Treatment options include extracting the hemorrhoid itself or extracting the clot and vein while under local anaesthetic.

Anal cracks

Another structural ailment is anal fissures. They are fissures or breaks in your anus's lining. The passage of very hard or wet faeces is the most frequent cause of an anal fissure. The underlying muscles that regulate the movement of stool through the anus and out of the body are visible due to the split in the anal lining. One of the worst conditions you might have is an anal fissure since the exposed muscles aggravate when they come into contact with air or faeces. After bowel motions, this causes excruciating searing pain, bleeding, or spasms.

Painkillers, dietary fiber to prevent the formation of big, thick stools, and sitz baths (sitting in a few inches of warm water) are the first treatments for anal fissures. Surgery to fix the fissure may be required if these remedies are ineffective in relieving your discomfort.

Perianal fistulas

Another structural illness known as perianal abscesses may develop from an infection brought on by blocked little anal glands that open within your anus due to the bacteria that is constantly present in these glands. An abscess forms when pus starts to form. The abscess is drained as part of the treatment, often at the doctor's office while under local anaesthetic.

A fistula anal

After an abscess is drained, an anal fistula—another structural illness—often develops. It's an odd tunnel that resembles a tube that leads from the anal canal to a skin hole close to the anus opening. Itching and irritation are caused by bodily wastes that are sent into your anal canal and out through the skin. Fistulas may also result in bleeding, discomfort, and drainage. Surgery is often required to "close off" the fistula and drain the abscess since they seldom heal on their own.

Distinctive illness

The condition known as diverticulosis is the existence of tiny protrusions, or diverticula, in the strong wall of your large intestine that develops in vulnerable intestinal regions. The sigmoid colon, the high-pressure region of the bottom large intestine, is where they often arise. In Western societies, 10% of persons over 40 and 50% of people over 60 have diverticular disease, which is a highly prevalent condition. It is often brought on by a diet lacking in roughage, or fiber. Diverticulitis may sometimes arise from or proceed from diverticulosis.

About 10% of patients with outpouchings have complications from diverticular illness. Among them include diverticulitis, an infection or inflammation of the pouches that may cause bleeding and blockage. When treating diverticulitis, one may also cure constipation and, in extreme cases, use antibiotics. In patients with severe problems, surgery is required as a last option to remove the affected diseased colonic section.

Malignancy and colon polyps
The second most prevalent kind of cancer diagnosed in the US each year is colorectal cancer, affecting 130,000 Americans. Fortunately, colorectal cancer is one of the most treatable types of the illness because of advancements in early

identification and treatment. Long before symptoms show up, the illness may be prevented, detected, and treated using a range of screening tests.

The significance of screening for colorectal cancer

Colon polyps, which are benign (non-cancerous) growths in the tissues lining your colon and rectum, are the precursor to almost all colorectal malignancies. When these polyps enlarge and aberrant cells begin to form and infiltrate the surrounding tissue, cancer is likely to occur. Colorectal cancer may be avoided by having polyps removed. During a colonoscopy screening, almost all precancerous polyps may be removed without causing any discomfort. Colon cancer has the potential to spread throughout the body if it is not detected in its early stages. More complex surgical approaches are needed for more advanced cancer.

Since the majority of early-stage colorectal cancers have no symptoms, screening is crucial. The cancer may be already well advanced when symptoms do appear. Abdominal discomfort, weight loss, constipation, narrowing of the stool, blood in or mixed with the stool, and persistent fatigue are some of the symptoms.

One of four methods is often used to detect colorectal cancer cases:

- by starting screenings for colorectal cancer in those at average risk at age 45.
- via screening individuals who are more likely to develop colorectal cancer (such as those who have a personal or family history of colon polyps or cancer).
- via examining the gut in those who have symptoms.
- unplanned discovery during a regular check-up.
- The greatest chance of a treatment is early discovery.

Chapter 2: Building a Foundation for Gut Health

2.1 The Role of Nutrition in Gut Health

The immune system and gut microbiota health depend on a good diet. While a bad diet may weaken the immune system and increase vulnerability to infections, a good, balanced diet and lifestyle can enhance our immune system. A varied diet that includes a range of foods will provide your body with the nutrition it needs to maintain a strong immune system.

Dietitians of Canada advise against using supplements and instead suggest obtaining your nutrition from diet. This is because food contains a variety of vitamins and minerals, protein, healthy fats, antioxidants, and other nutrients that are critical to the immune system's correct operation.

Food sources and the function of nutrients

White blood cells, which are essential for immunological response and control, form normally with the help of vitamin A, which helps the immune system work normally. Vitamin A-rich foods include colourful fruits and vegetables including broccoli, kale, and spinach as well as red bell peppers, tomatoes, melon, and mango.

Vitamin B6 (pyridoxine) is necessary for the immune system to operate normally and is needed as a coenzyme for the metabolism of cytokines and antibodies, which are substances produced by immune cells. Fish, poultry, beef, potatoes, and beans are examples of good dietary sources.

Vitamin B9, also known as folic acid or folate, is essential for the immune system's development and proliferation of T cells, which the body needs to fend off infections. Whereas folate is present in food, folic acid is found in vitamin supplements. The following foods include folate: cooked dry beans, peas, and lentils; fruits (banana, raspberries, grapefruit, and cantaloupe); enriched grain products (bread, cereals, pasta); spinach, asparagus, romaine lettuce, beets, and broccoli.

Because it is necessary for the synthesis of proteins and DNA, vitamin B12 has an impact on the immune system. It also plays a function in the development of new immune cells and antibodies. The greatest foods to consume to get vitamin B12 include fish, poultry, eggs, dairy products, and lean meats.

Because of its antioxidant qualities, vitamin C helps the immune system and immunological response operate normally. A wide variety of fruits and vegetables contain vitamin C. For a midday snack, try raw peppers or cooked broccoli, or have a ½ cup of strawberries for dessert. You could even have a glass of orange juice or grapefruit for breakfast!

Vitamin D is necessary for the immune system to operate properly and is crucial for controlling the generation of antibodies and inflammatory reactions. Some foods do contain vitamin D, although not many do, such as margarine and cow's milk. egg yolks, fatty fish (sardines and salmon), and fortified orange juice. Go to Unlock Food for further information about vitamin D.

Silver is essential for the production and proper operation of immune cells and helps the immune system operate normally. Foods heavy in protein, such as oysters, cattle, pig, cheese (cheddar, swiss, gouda, brie, mozzarella), turkey, baked beans, and tinned lentils, are good sources of zinc.

The synthesis of cytokines, which are substances produced by immune cells, and the proper operation of T lymphocytes, which are necessary to defend the body against infections, depend on iron for healthy immune function. A wide range of plant foods, animal meals, and iron-fortified goods (such as bread, pasta, and cereals) contain iron. Beef, pig, chicken, lamb, liver, kidney, oysters, shrimp, octopus, chicken, duck, quail, mackerel, trout, bass, and tuna fish are a few examples of particular cuisine.

Immune cells need copper to produce energy and to defend themselves from oxidative damage. Shellfish, nuts and seeds, oysters, unsweetened baking chocolate, beef, and liver are food sources of copper.

Mineral selenium has a significant impact on the immune system and is associated with a rise in T cells, which are necessary to defend the body against infections. Foods including oysters, liver, tuna in cans, roasted pork, eggs, brazil nuts, and more contain it.

Remembering that more isn't always better is crucial. No proof consuming more of a nutrient than what our bodies need can boost immunity.

The phrase "boosting the immune function" is untrue.

Because the gut microbiota strives to preserve its homeostasis or balance, you may not necessarily want your immune system to be functioning at above-average levels.

Consult a qualified dietician if you have questions about your nutritional consumption or believe you may need a supplement. It is advisable to consult your physician before beginning any supplement regimen. Excessive doses of zinc and selenium may be poisonous, and consuming more than 2,000 mg of vitamin C daily might cause adverse effects including diarrhoea.

Eating a wide range of meals and maintaining a healthy, balanced lifestyle are the goals. The more varied the food, the more diversified the microbiota, and it also provides a broad range of nutrients. The American Gut Project's findings show that a diet richer in plant varieties is linked to a more diverse gut microbiota, and gut microbial diversity is a key sign of both gut health and general health. In a reexamination, scientists also found that when it comes to the gut microbiota, it is critical to consider the diet as its whole rather than focusing on specific items. Particularly, higher microbial diversity was linked to a flexitarian eating pattern. Microbiota variety is also associated with flexitarian diets, such as the Mediterranean diet.

However, some food kinds and ingredients may be especially beneficial as they support the protection of the gut barrier and the growth and strengthening of the gut microbiota.

Foods that are fermented and contain living cultures, such as yogurt, kimchi, sauerkraut, and kefir, may contribute to the gut microbiota's increased variety.

Certain probiotic-containing fermented foods, such as kefir and certain probiotic yogurt, may also help maintain a healthy gut microbiome.

Prebiotics support the development of good bacteria in the gut and strengthen the gut barrier. Some of these microorganisms are forms of dietary fiber that may be found in fruit and vegetables or concentrated in supplements.

In conclusion, a rich, varied diet that includes a range of foods—such as certain fermented foods, probiotics, and prebiotics—is crucial for meeting our dietary requirements and promoting the healthy operation of the immune system and gut microbiota.

2.2 Hydration and Its Impact on Digestion

One of the most crucial elements in enhancing gut health and digestion is staying hydrated. Whether you drink your water hot or cold makes no difference. Water may help the body transport nutrients around and eliminate waste and other pollutants, regardless of its temperature. In addition, a hydrated stomach aids in improved skin, less inflammation, and regularity of bowel movements. But how does hydration function?

How is gut health enhanced by maintaining hydration?

helps avoid constipation
To facilitate the passage of food through your stomach, intestines, and colon, your body draws fluids to the digestive system. Food may get trapped or slow down if there is not enough fluid to keep it flowing, which may result in bloating or constipation.

Envision yourself sliding down a waterslide at a theme park. You get caught and have to carefully make your way down the slide if there isn't enough water to push you down. This is comparable to the effects of dehydration on the faeces in your stomach.

Aids in food digestion by breaking it down

In the small intestine, fluid is utilized to carry the acids and enzymes that break down food. Imagine it as a kind of vehicle that returns to the bloodstream after dropping off the deconstruction crew and picking up the nutrients.

reduces gastrointestinal inflammation

It is more difficult for food to get through your digestive system when you are dehydrated. Your intestines may become inflamed in some areas due to the continuous friction of food in the absence of fluid transportation. This discomfort may eventually cause the gut's inflammation to rise.

lowers the chance of a leaky gut

How does your stomach become porous? You may be familiar with the phrase "leaky gut" to refer to the permeability of the gut. When the gut walls' tight connections loosen, this occurs.

This looseness makes it possible for dangerous elements to enter your circulation, including germs, poisons, and leftover food particles. Your intestinal walls may become more porous if the inflammation in your gut lining lasts too long. Being well-hydrated lowers intestinal inflammation, which lowers the likelihood of gut permeability.

How can you determine your level of hydration?

You don't experience thirst. We just need to learn to listen to your body, which is quite adept at letting you know precisely what you need when you need it. You're probably already dehydrated if you're experiencing thirst.

You have colourless or very light yellow urine. Your urine will take on a deeper, more golden hue as you grow dehydrated. You should drink extra water if your pee is black!

How to Stay Hydrated:
- Alcohol and caffeine increase dehydration, so cut down on your intake of these substances.
- Before meals, just before bed, and as soon as you wake up, have a glass of water.
- "Eat your water" by munching on foods like watermelon, strawberries, cantaloupe, celery, and spinach that are rich in water content. These meals may help you improve your hydration intake since they contain 90% water.
- Always have a bottle of water with you. You will be motivated to drink more water throughout the day by the continual reminder of the bottle in front of you.

You don't like the flavour of water. Not an issue! To add some taste, try experimenting with adding fresh fruits and veggies like cucumbers, lemons, and strawberries. For hot summer days, you may also add frozen blueberries to the ice cubes.

2.3 Balancing Gut Health with Lifestyle Choices

It is healthy to be a part of an engaged culture. But eating Greek yogurt as a snack is not the only way to improve your gut health. Your lifestyle choices, including exercise, sleep, mindfulness, meditation, and other activities, are just as important to your health as what you eat.

Further evidence of the connection between gut microbiota health and mental health is emerging as the gut-brain axis study progresses. The population of microscopic organisms that inhabit the gastrointestinal tract—also known as the gut—is reflected in the gut microbiome. The creation of neurotransmitters, including serotonin, epinephrine, dopamine, and norepinephrine, depends on the environment in the gut, which is maintained in part by this community. Behaviour, mood, and stress reactions are all regulated by neurotransmitters.

However, our lifestyle and mental health have an impact on how well our gut works. The gut microbiota may suffer, for instance, from sleep deprivation or living in a stressful environment. Ten instances of how good lifestyle choices impact the composition and balance of the gut microbiota are shown below.

Ten Easy Lifestyle Changes to Promote Gut Health:

1.For ten minutes a day, meditate to help your body and mind relax. The gut microbiota is negatively impacted by stress, and practices like mindfulness and meditation may help lower stress and promote gut health.

2.To promote good sleep, sleep in a room that is between 64° and 69° F (17.8° and 20.6° C). Lack of sleep may lead to many health issues and have a detrimental effect on the ratios of gut flora.

3.Steer clear of opioids and/or anti-inflammatory medications (where feasible). The gut flora may suffer from overuse of opioids and/or anti-inflammatory medications.

4.Steer clear of processed carbs and concentrate on sources of carbs high in nutrients. Vegetable-based carbohydrates are good for the variety and general health of the gut microbiota.

5.For the following eight weeks, try to limit or eliminate alcohol intake to no more than two drinks each week. Excessive alcohol use may have a deleterious effect on the diversity of the gut microbiome.

6.To aid in digestion and prevent dehydration, increase your intake of water and other fluids based on how thirsty you are.

7.Limit your intake of caffeine to one or two cups before midday and cut down on the amount of goods that contain it. While excessive coffee drinking may lead to dehydration, irregular digestion, and sleep difficulties, it can also have a positive impact on the microbiota.

8.Make an effort to eat a range of meals high in protein. The greatest source of protein is whole foods, but if you need to reach your protein targets, it might be helpful to add in an additional protein shake. Amino acids, which make up protein, are used by the gut flora to create vital metabolites like indole-3-propionic acid, which might promote overall health and well-being.

9.Weekly self- or professional massages may promote the creation of neurotransmitters such as serotonin, which is involved in supporting the gut-brain link.

10.Vitamin synthesis is beneficial by spending at least 10 minutes each day in direct sunshine, which supports the health of the gut microbiota. If you live somewhere with little to no sun exposure, you may want to discuss vitamin D3 supplements with your doctor.

The diversity and well-being of the gut microbiome may be significantly impacted by modest lifestyle modifications. Numerous facets of your general well-being, such as immune function, digestion, illness prevention, sleep quality, and much more, are correlated with gut health. Even one of these lifestyle changes may improve your general well-being and the composition of your gut flora.

Chapter 3: A Healthy Gut Diet

3.1 Foods to Avoid for Optimal Gut Health

Maintaining intestinal health requires sensible food selection. To greatly enhance your digestive health, we've put up a list of the top 10 items that you should stay away from.

1. Processed meals

The gut microbiota may be harmed by processed meals since they are heavy in harmful fats, preservatives, and additives.

2. Pure sugar

The equilibrium of microorganisms in your stomach may be upset by refined sugar, which can cause inflammation and digestive problems.

3. Gluten: Gluten is a protein present in wheat, barley, and rye that may irritate the gastrointestinal tract in those who have gluten sensitivity but do not have celiac disease.

4. Milk-based goods
Dairy products may trigger digestive problems including gas, bloating, and diarrhoea in a lot of individuals.

5. Fried cuisine
Fried meals include a lot of bad fats, which may damage your gut flora and cause inflammation.

6. flesh from red flesh
Eating red meat regularly raises the risk of colon cancer and may cause inflammation.

7. Synthetic sweeteners
Artificial sweeteners have the potential to upset your gut's bacterial balance and aggravate digestive problems.

8. Tobacco

Drinking too much alcohol may damage your gut microbiota, which can cause immune system decline and digestive problems.

9. Espresso

While a reasonable amount of caffeine is usually harmless, too much of it may lead to stomach problems including acid reflux and heartburn.

10. Corn syrup with high fructose

High-fructose corn syrup is a highly processed sugar that may cause inflammation and upset your gut's bacterial balance.

Foods to Eat to Maintain Gut Health

These are some dietary choices that support intestinal health.

foods high in fiber. Whole grains, fruits, and vegetables are examples of foods rich in fiber that may support the health of the gut microbiota.

fermented food items. Yogurt, kefir, and kimchi are examples of fermented foods that contain good bacteria that may maintain a balanced gut microbiota.

Prebiotics. Probiotics are good bacteria that may assist in enhancing digestive health and balance your gut microbiota.
beneficial fats. Nuts, avocados, and olive oil are among the foods rich in good fats that may support intestinal health.

3.2 Meal Ideas for a healthy gut

Gut health may be complicated; an imbalanced microbiota can lead to a variety of issues, such as insomnia and poor digestion. With so many gut-healthy ingredients in these high-fiber recipes—like beans, broccoli, and apples—you can have something tasty and healthful to finish your day in only thirty minutes. You may enjoy great and easy recipes like our Seared Scallops with Green Goddess Slaw and White Bean and sun-dried Tomato Gnocchi each night of the week.

Pasta with Garlic-Anchovies and Broccolini

Here, we add some crumbled goat cheese to the last pasta dish to give it a wonderful, acidic taste. However, you may also add cheese and the remaining boiling water to the pasta in Step 3 if you would rather have a creamy sauce.

Sun-Dried Tomato & White Bean Gnocchi

The key ingredient in this dish is the sun-dried tomatoes, which provide umami and texture. They give this meal an excellent source of vitamins C and K when combined with the spinach.

Pasta with Crispy Pancetta, Spinach, and Lima Beans

Fresh spinach spaghetti is our choice since it cooks fast and offers a vibrant splash of colour. Lima beans gain flavour when cooked with pancetta drippings.

Cream Cheese and Creamy White Chili

Canned white beans and quick-cooking chicken thighs make this rich yet healthful white chicken chilli come together quickly. When your soups don't have a lengthy simmer period, mashing part of the beans helps to quickly thicken the liquid. The last amount of richness and a touch of the sweet tang is added by cream cheese.

Green Goddess Slaw with Seared Scallops

The herbaceous dressing that coats this salad is made creamier by the addition of avocado, yogurt, and buttermilk.

Lima bean and orange-mint freekeh salad

There are so many vibrant vegetables in this salad: oranges, snap peas, radishes, and fresh mint. Slice the snap peas into long, thin strips for visually appealing slices.

Soup with White Beans and Pasta

To flavor this soup, we utilize a mixture of onions, celery, and carrots called mirepoix. To make sure you always have some on hand without having to worry about it going bad, put a bag of the mixture that you got at the shop in your freezer.

Slaw & Black Bean Bagel

This simple open-face sandwich recipe calls for a jalapeño-Cheddar bagel, but you could instead use a plain bagel. For a filling snack, top half of a bagel with fresh slaw and black beans.

Wraps of black beans, greens, and cilantro vinaigrette

These easy-to-make wraps are bursting with vibrant cilantro flavor thanks to a simple salad dressed with a zesty vinaigrette. Mashed beans and avocado go nicely with the mix; they bind everything together.

Bowl of Black Beans with Cauliflower "Rice"

Bowl of Black Beans with Cauliflower "Rice"

This flavorful rice dish made with cauliflower just takes a few minutes to prepare and serves one person. In addition to cutting down on carbs, using frozen riced cauliflower instead of rice expedites preparation.

Curry with Vegan Coconut Chickpeas

Purchase precut vegetables from the grocery store's salad bar to expedite the preparation of this 20-minute vegan curry. Serve over cooked brown rice for a hearty, filling supper. If you want to keep this vegan, seek for simmer sauces that have 400 mg or less of salt and check the ingredient list for cream or fish sauce. Add a few dashes of your preferred hot sauce at the end if you want a spicy kick.

Chapter 4: Lifestyle Practices for a Healthy Gut

4.1 Stress Management and Gut Health

Your body's reaction to certain stimuli, which might originate from perceived, social, environmental, or physical causes, is called stress. Numerous intricate brain connections that impact bodily processes outside of your conscious awareness are involved in the stress response. Stress has a major role in digestive health and wellness because the enteric nervous system (enteric tract) contains more neurons than the spinal cord—more than one hundred million in total.

Stress-related physiological changes include:

- An increased level of consciousness rapid respiration and heart rate
- Increased blood pressure and a spike in cholesterol levels
- A rise in tenseness in the muscles

This booklet contains advice for those who, although generally well-functioning in society, may sometimes find it difficult to handle everyday stressors. You should get treatment from a trained medical professional if you have a mood condition, such as bipolar disorder, clinical depression, or anxiety disorder.

Stress may help you perform better because short bursts of stress prepare your body to work harder and more intensively. As long as the tension passes and your body swiftly returns to normal, this "fight or flight" reaction may be useful for brief spikes in energy and focus.

While some people cope with significant upheavals without a second thought, others become disturbed at even the smallest change in their daily routine. The majority of folks fall in the middle. It's crucial to keep in mind that stress may be beneficial in moderation. It might be the inspiration you need to push yourself to your limits and maintain your attention and alertness. Stress only becomes problematic when it is unchecked or persistent.

Although each person experiences stress in different ways, there is a genuine risk to your relationships, mental stability, and physical health.

Effects on the Body

Persistent stress induces an additional level of physiological reaction in people who encounter it. This response includes decreased immune system performance, continuous elevation of blood pressure and cholesterol, increased creation of stomach acid, and decreased levels of sex hormones. Normal life stresses might become too much to handle in this scenario. A person experiencing stress may have physical symptoms when little stressors, such as changes in personal relationships, professional obstacles, family issues, or financial hardships, accumulate.

Stress in all its forms may affect the body by escalating pre-existing problems or bringing on physical symptoms such as headaches, tense muscles, lack of desire for sexual activity, constipation or diarrhea, sleeplessness, and changes in appetite.

Effects Specific to GI

Should you suffer from a gastrointestinal (GI) sickness or problem, you might be more susceptible to the negative impact of stress on your current condition, which could lead to worsening of symptoms, acceleration of the disease progression, and disruption of the healing process. Although psychological stress may exacerbate pre-existing illnesses or raise the risk of recurrence in those with dormant disease, research has not shown that stress causes structural issues in the gastrointestinal tract. There is evidence of this for inflammatory bowel illnesses (Crohn's and ulcerative colitis) as well as functional gastrointestinal disorders (IBS, dyspepsia, GERD, hypertension).

A person who struggles to manage long-term stress maintains an overactive condition in their body, which interferes with regular bodily functions, including the digestive system. Physical manifestations include immune system suppression, increased muscular tension, and a blood shift flow away from the gastrointestinal tract. For those with gastrointestinal disorders, these modifications are important.

Supervisory

Reducing your stress levels and developing useful stress-reduction strategies may improve your prognosis for the illness and lessen the intensity of your gastrointestinal symptoms.

Here are a few useful tips for stress management.

*Consume a balanced diet according to Health . The secret to excellent physical and mental health is proper eating. Your body experiences more stress and is less able to recover from malnutrition. Your body will appreciate you for making sensible eating choices in addition to lowering stress levels!

*Learn to breathe from your belly more slowly and deeply to improve your breathing technique. If you don't intentionally try to breathe deeply, your body won't obtain enough oxygen to completely relax since stress may lead to shallow breathing.

*Keep an eye on your "self-talk" since a lot of anxiety is self-induced, which means we often talk ourselves into thinking about the worst-case situations or exaggerating little instances.

*Track how frequently you worry about things like making errors or losing your career by keeping an eye on your negative thoughts. Make an effort to replace every pessimistic notion with a realistically optimistic one.

Get moving, since physical activity is a well-known way to relieve stress. Make sure to gradually increase your workout regimen while monitoring your body's tolerance. However, proceed with care, since those suffering from ulcerative colitis, Crohn's disease, hiatus hernia, or gastroesophageal reflux disease (GERD) may find their gastrointestinal symptoms worsened by high-impact workouts.

*To stop time from managing you, improve your time management skills. We often misjudge how much work a task will need, which causes us to be late. To have a better understanding of how long certain chores truly take, try maintaining a time management record for a week.

*When the time is right, learn when to say no. Feeling that you can "do it all" puts undue strain on yourself. Develop your ability to create personal limits. Refuse to take on more tasks or duties for which you lack the necessary time or energy in a kind but firm manner.

*Take some time for yourself; otherwise, our overactive nervous systems will continue to function at full speed into the next day. Our bodies and brains need variation. Every week, try to set aside at least one day to do something you really like, like reading, watching TV, or just hanging out with friends.

*Enjoy a big belly laugh as this all-natural stress reliever helps to ease muscular tension, decrease blood pressure, and calm breathing and heart rate.

If you think you need more assistance than what the aforementioned tactics can provide, seek professional aid. Expert psychologists have created a variety of strategies and practical resources to assist people in managing stress better. Treatment techniques that are more commonly employed include deep breathing exercises, biofeedback, hypnosis, progressive muscle relaxation training, time management techniques, lifestyle modifications, cognitive behavioral therapy, assertiveness training, deep breathing exercises, systematic desensitization, and brief psychotherapy.

When using stress management services, proceed with caution to make sure the person treating you is properly qualified and licensed. A therapist with inadequate training may treat you ineffectively, waste your time and money, miss more significant issues, and/or finally make you stop seeking professional help. Basic healthcare plans cover several programs in many locations, while some extended healthcare policies include extra therapies. Request a referral from your doctor to certain local services.

4.2 Exercise and Its Impact on Digestion

Your body doesn't use energy for digestion while you work out. Rather, it reduces the speed at which digestion is happening to maximize blood flow to your lungs and muscles. As a result, digestion and activity are incompatible.

Because the demand is not as pressing when you're fit, less blood is drawn from your digestive system. Being in shape increases the efficiency of your muscles. Your digestive system may get stronger with regular exercise, which can enhance intestinal motility and excretion over time.

Consumption and Activity

Give your body enough time to process before working out. You could require a few hours to fully digest a meal that is high in fats and proteins. Your blood sugar increases during food digestion to aid in the process. To focus all of your efforts on your exercise, I advise waiting for it to return to normal.

It's important to drink enough water while working out. While exercising, dehydration may lead to GI issues including acid reflux and constipation. Additionally, when we are dehydrated, our intestines may have trouble adequately absorbing the nutrients from the food we eat, which in some situations might result in malnutrition.

Exercise and some gastrointestinal conditions
We've long known that regular exercise is good for your general health. Exercise may affect a variety of gastrointestinal disorders due to its impact on your immune system and the release of endorphins into your body, which occur naturally during exercise.

Exercise relieves constipation by speeding up the normal contraction of the intestinal muscles, which reduces the amount of time food takes to pass through the large intestine. It is simpler for the feces to pass out of the body when the quantity of water it absorbs is reduced.

GERD: It's crucial to consider when to exercise in relation to mealtimes. My advice is to wait two hours after a meal before exercising to reduce the likelihood of reflux occurring when the stomach is full.

Diverticular Disease: People with sedentary jobs, such as sitting at a desk, are more likely to develop diverticular disease. Frequent exercise may speed up food transit through the GI tract, lower colonic pressure, and encourage bowel movements. A decreased risk of complications related to diverticular illness is linked to all three of these findings. Exercise also helps reduce chronic pain and discomfort in the belly by releasing natural endorphins.

Colon Cancer: According to a 2009 research by the National Health Institute, the most physically active people had a 24% reduced risk of colon cancer than the least physically active people. The study looked at the relationship between physical activity and colon cancer risk.

Workout to Promote Better Digestive Health
We should all exercise for a variety of reasons, including improved immune system function, more frequent bowel movements, a more diversified and healthier gut microbiome, lowered risk of colon cancer, and enhanced gut motility. Intriguing research findings such as this one also exist to support that assertion:

Men's rugby players and male non-athletes were the subjects of a 2016 National University of Ireland research, which found that the athletes' gut microbiomes were much more diverse. Additionally, there were more Akkermansiaceae bacteria in the gut flora of the rugby players, which is known to reduce systemic inflammation.

It should be equally obvious that regular exercise also helps with stress relief, maintaining a healthy weight, which helps with problems like fatty liver, diabetes, and heart disease, and boosting energy levels throughout the day. I am aware that many of us have very busy lives and that there are several (what I like to term, excuses) for why it is difficult to exercise. You must decide for yourself if fitting exercise into your hectic schedule a few times a week for thirty minutes or so is worth the investment in your physical well-being. It could lead to a longer and better life for you.

4.3 Sleep, Circadian Rhythms, and Gut Health

The connection between circadian rhythms, meal timing, and metabolic health is known as chrono-nutrition. The enormous influence of circadian rhythms on the host's metabolic processes and gut flora has led to a recent surge in interest in this area of nutrition. The term "circadian rhythms" describes a set of natural oscillators that connect internal physiological processes to the outside world. These oscillators are produced by circadian biological clocks.

A significant amount of the overall makeup of the gut microbiota varies rhythmically over the day. Furthermore, via many signaling mechanisms, the gut microbiota synchronizes the host's circadian biological clocks. These findings suggest that host circadian rhythms and gut bacteria may interact and that food timing and patterns may be important factors in this interaction.

Diet, circadian cycles, and gut microbiome interactions
The time, frequency, and regularity of meals, as well as the quality of the food, all contribute to the regulation of the interaction between gut microbiota and circadian rhythms.

When to eat

The light-dark cycle of the sun controls the brain's fundamental circadian clock. Peripheral circadian clocks in the liver, pancreas, and gastrointestinal (GI) tract, however, are mostly synchronized by food components since they are not directly exposed to light.

Research has shown that eating in the late evening may change hormone release and interfere with circadian rhythms (a condition known as chrono-disturbance). Furthermore, it has been shown that a 1-hour increase in the last meal time of the day is linked to changes in metabolism, such as elevated C-reactive protein, decreased high-density lipoprotein (good cholesterol), and worsened glycemic control and body weight regulation.

Time-restricted eating is the practice of consuming a certain quantity of food within a predetermined window of time. It has been discovered that this specific eating pattern modifies the makeup of the gut microbiota, including the induction of helpful bacterial communities and the decrease of detrimental bacterial populations. It is thought that limiting food access time in this way mimics circadian rhythm-based natural eating behaviors.

Regularity and frequency of meals

Eating irregularities have been shown to desynchronize the central and peripheral circadian clocks, which modifies circadian cycles. Those who eat well in the evening are far more likely to forego breakfast, lunch, or midmorning snacks, according to several research.

Higher food consumption is associated with less dangerous bacterial populations in the gut, according to research done on horses. Nevertheless, no research has looked at how regularity and frequency of meals affect the microbiota of the human stomach.

Diet standard

The body's innate propensity to be awake or sleeping at certain periods of the day is known as a chronotype. There is evidence that a person's diet quality may be influenced by their chronotype.

Studies have shown that late-evening eaters consume more sugar regularly than morning eaters, although chronotypes do not seem to have an impact on the consumption of macro- and micronutrients. Furthermore, a few studies have linked unhealthy or low-quality diets to eating patterns in the evening.

With several health advantages, the Mediterranean diet is regarded as one of the greatest eating regimens. It is well recognized that this diet lowers the risk of metabolic and cardiovascular illnesses, as well as all-cause morbidity and death. Research has shown that individuals with a morning chronotype tend to follow the Mediterranean diet more closely and control their weight more well.

Studies on the link between gut microbiota, circadian rhythms, and food quality have shown that high-fat diets change the chronobiology of the gut microbiota, which affects the synthesis of microbial metabolites and impairs circadian rhythms and metabolism.

Diet, gut microbiota, and circadian rhythm crosstalk's effects on health
Numerous chronic illnesses, such as mental health issues, malignancies, and metabolic and cardiovascular diseases, are linked to gut microbiota dysbiosis and diet-related chrono-disruption.

There is evidence that a changed cardiometabolic profile is linked to an evening chronotype. Among those who eat in the evening, there has been a notable change in the rhythmicity of the gut microbiota and the metabolism of fats and carbohydrates.

Additionally, studies have linked the evening chronotype to an increased risk of colon, lung, prostate, and breast malignancies. It has been proposed that circadian disturbance modifies the sleep cycle and cell proliferation, hence raising the risk of cancer. By altering the synthesis of metabolites produced by gut microbes, such as bile acids and short-chain fatty acids (SCFA), circadian abnormalities may also accelerate the development of cancer.

A dysbiosis of the gut microbiota and circadian rhythm may raise the likelihood of depression and other mental illnesses. The altered rhythmicity of neurotransmitters linked to mood regulation may be the cause of this.

Recent research indicates that circadian rhythms may be altered by a greater abundance of pro-inflammatory and a lower abundance of SCFA-producing microbial communities, both of which increase the risk of depression.

4.4 The Gut-Brain Connection

There is a serious connection between the gut and the brain; worry may cause stomach issues and vice versa. Have you ever encountered anything "gut-wrenching"? Are there circumstances that cause you to "feel nauseous"? Have you ever had stomach butterflies"? There's a reason we use these idioms. Emotions may affect the digestive system. Feelings such as anger, worry, grief, and exhilaration, among others, may set off sensations in the stomach.

The stomach and intestines are directly impacted by the brain. For example, just thinking about eating might cause the stomach's contents to flow out before the meal does. This relationship is reciprocal. Both a disturbed brain and a troublesome intestine may communicate with one another via signals. As a result, worry, stress, or depression may either induce or result from a person's stomach or intestinal problems. This is due to the close connection that exists between the brain and the gastrointestinal (GI) system.

This is particularly true when someone has unsettled stomach symptoms without a clear medical reason. It is difficult to attempt gut healing for these functional GI illnesses without taking stress and emotion into account.

Your gut speaks to your brain and your brain responds. You've encountered this communication if you've ever had a "gut feeling." It's similar to how picturing an exciting occasion may give you butterflies in your stomach while seeing something horrible can give you the chills. And it's about how you can make decisions based on your gut instinct, or "going with your gut."

Nerves (your nervous system) allow your brain to interact with every part of your body. However, your gut and intellect are like best friends. They discuss a wide range of topics, from emotional to realistic and bodily. More data than any other system in the body is transferred between the stomach and the brain. Your stomach contains more nerve cells than any other place in your body, save your brain.

What does the gut-brain link serve to accomplish?

Together, our digestive tracts and brains have developed to help us live. Our diets are very important to our general health and have changed significantly throughout time based on what was available. For us to ensure that we were getting the nutrients we needed, our stomachs and brains had to work together closely. We also required a reliable alert system in case we ate the incorrect food or had to stop our digestion.

Your brain's emotional center is a component of this alarm system. Your emotional brain takes over after a physical injury to remind you to prevent that harm in the future. Your gut's physical feelings may appear more strong while you're feeling emotional. Your stress levels and emotional reactions may also be elevated by intense physical sensations. There is a very powerful feedback loop between your stomach and brain.

Which bodily systems are impacted by the gut-brain connection?

Research indicates that the interplay between your stomach and brain might affect your:

- Desire and fullness.
- Cravings and preferences for food.
- Dietary intolerances and sensitivities.
- The movement of muscles in the Gut
- Breakdown
- Digestion
- Feeling
- Activism
- Tension levels
- pain sensitivity
- mental operations
- Autonomy

The digestive tract and brain are connected by a network of nerves called the gut-brain axis, which medical professionals use to describe this signaling network. However, the endocrine system—which creates hormones that convey emotions like stress, hunger, and fullness—and the neurological system are tightly related. Furthermore, it collaborates closely with your immune system to help your stomach heal and recover from injuries and illnesses.

Among the important participants in the gut-brain link within this network are:

Nervous system of the stomach
The neural network that acts within your gastrointestinal (GI) tract and regulates digestion is known as your enteric nervous system. The most intricate neural network outside of your brain, with over 500 million neurons. It is also distinct in that it has some degree of autonomy from your central nervous system and brain. Its status has prompted some scientists to call it a "second brain."

Your autonomic nervous system, which controls the automatic operations of your internal organs, has an additional branch called the enteric nervous system. It functions both independently and as a component of your whole autonomic nerve system. It can collect data on the state of your GI tract, interpret that data locally, and provide a response without relaying that data back to your brain.

Sacral Nerve

The primary nerve that connects your brain to your enteric nervous system is the vagus nerve. It is one of the twelve cranial nerves, which start in the skull and branch out as they pass through the body. Your vagus nerve transmits sensory data from your enteric nervous system to your brain about the circumstances within your stomach. It responds by sending motor impulses from your brain to your stomach.

Your gut's reflexes in reaction to changing circumstances, such as chemical shifts or the presence of food, are mediated by the vagus nerve. We refer to them as vagal reflexes. Your enteric nervous system regulates intrinsic vagal reflexes independently of the brain. Your enteric and central nervous systems communicate with one another to control extrinsic reflexes.

Stomach microbiota

Unbelievably, the gut-brain link is also influenced by the microorganisms that reside there. Many of the chemical neurotransmitters that transfer information between your stomach and brain are produced by or assisted by gut microorganisms. They also create additional compounds that enter your system and have an impact on your brain. Your stomach and brain may change the environment in your gut, which in turn can impact your gut microbiota.

According to recent research, some neurological, mental health, and functional gastrointestinal diseases may be influenced by the gut microbiota. When there is no apparent medical basis for a chronic set of symptoms, the condition is considered functional. People with mental health illnesses like anxiety and those with functional gastrointestinal diseases like IBS (irritable bowel syndrome) have a lot of similarities.

4.5 Holistic Approaches to Gut Health

Your gut's health is influenced by physical, emotional, and mental variables, much like any other system in the body. We go over how to approach your gut health from a whole-person perspective in this holistic guide to gut health, which takes into account your mind, body, and emotions.

1. Enhance Your Nutrition
Enhancing your nutrition is one of the first steps in achieving comprehensive gut health. Typically, this indicates:

- Determine the triggers and allergies in food
- Cutting less on processed items in your diet Lower your intake of sugars and refined carbs
- Boost your diet's natural fiber intake.
- Give organic, grass-fed meats priority.

- Consume a lot of fruits and veggies.
- Include fermented foods like sauerkraut, kimchi, and kefir in your diet.
- Examine your digestive system to see whether you are producing enough HCl and enzymes to break down meals.

Your diet should be optimized to make sure your body gets the nutrients it needs, minimize pollutants, stay away from items that cause inflammation, and maintain a balanced microbiota.

2-Repair and Maintain Your Microbiota

Eating a nutritious, well-balanced diet maintains your microbiome at its best most of the time. Probiotics may, however, be beneficial in some situations. These include recuperating from bad eating habits, having medical conditions that limit your ability to absorb certain nutrients, having leaky gut syndrome, or having recently taken antibiotics.

Make sure the probiotics you choose to include in your diet are low in sugar since sugar may encourage the growth of candida in the digestive tract. Consult your holistic healthcare practitioner if you're thinking about including probiotics in your diet or if you're not sure which ones to take into account.

3. Minimize Inflammation

Chronic inflammation is another factor that leads to poor gut health. Chronic inflammation may harm healthy tissues, impair nutrition absorption, and create a leaky gut. It can also be brought on by underlying illnesses, stress, or allergies. Your body may be rebalanced and inflammation can be decreased by:

- Recognizing your dietary sensitivities or allergies and eliminating such items from your diet
- Avoiding highly processed or inflammatory foods like gluten
- Finding and treating underlying illnesses, including yeast or sinus infections

4-Enhance Stress Reduction
Your gut health is influenced by physical causes, but real holistic gut health also takes mental health into account. This is due to a gut-brain connection that establishes a relationship between your mental and digestive health. Extended or severe stress may have detrimental effects on your general well-being. This is because long-term stress may lower immunity and increase inflammation in the body. Because of this, stress reduction is a crucial component of overall gut health. To reduce stress, think about:

Yogic meditation
Taking Stress Reduction Exercise
Increasing the quality of sleep

5- Drink water
It's also critical to maintain enough hydration for overall intestinal health. In addition to being crucial for proper digestion, water also affects cell health, heals leaky gut, and boosts immunity. Drink half of your body weight in pounds in fluid ounces each day as a general guideline.

6-Eat Cautiously

It's crucial to develop the practice of mindful eating. This may guarantee that you're chewing your meal correctly and assist in avoiding overindulging. Furthermore, you should attempt to avoid eating while you're anxious since your body isn't as prepared to process food well when it's in the fight-or-flight response.

Chapter 5:Working with Healthcare Professionals

Although improving your gut health is a personal journey, there may be occasions when you need the advice and knowledge of medical specialists. This chapter will cover when and how to work with medical professionals to address particular gut health concerns and make sure you're headed in the correct direction for a fulfilling life.

Knowing When to Get Expert Assistance

Understanding the warning signals of when to seek medical advice is crucial before you can collaborate with them efficiently. These indicators might be:

Consistent Digestive Symptoms: It's time to see a doctor if you're dealing with ongoing digestive problems, such as persistent bloating, diarrhea, constipation, or unexplained weight loss.

Family History: Early intervention may be essential if you have a family history of gastrointestinal disorders, which may raise your risk.

Change in Bowel Habits: You should never disregard sudden or inexplicable changes in your bowel habits, such as the presence of blood in your stool.

Unexplained discomfort: If you have severe or persistent stomach discomfort for which there is no apparent reason, you should see a doctor.

Concerning symptoms: You shouldn't ignore symptoms that worry you, no matter how little they may seem.

Selecting the Appropriate Medical Expert

Concerns about gut health may be addressed by a variety of medical specialists. Selecting the appropriate one may have a big impact on your journey

Primary Care Physician: Usually, your first point of contact is your family physician. They can assist in diagnosing common digestive health problems and, if necessary, refer you to experts.

Gastroenterologists are experts in the diagnosis and treatment of a broad variety of gut-related disorders. They concentrate on the digestive system.

Registered Dietitian: A registered dietitian may provide customized nutrition guidance and meal planning if dietary changes are a major component of your gut health journey.

Functional Medicine Practitioner: To treat gut health holistically, these practitioners take into account the interplay between hereditary, environmental, and lifestyle variables.

Mental Health Professional: A mental health professional may assist in managing the psychological components of gut-brain connections, such as stress and irritable bowel syndrome (IBS).

Getting Ready for Your Medical Appointment

Take into consideration the following advice to get the most out of your medical appointments:

Maintain a Symptom Diary: Keep track of your symptoms, how long they last, and any trends or triggers you've seen.

Make a list of the queries and worries you would want to address with your healthcare professional. This makes sure you obtain the data you need.

Share Your Lifestyle: Your food, exercise routine, stress level, and sleep habits are all important for your healthcare practitioner to know to understand your overall health.

Please bring copies of any pertinent medical documents, especially results from any previous gastrointestinal tests, if you have had any previous testing.

Working together with medical experts is a collaboration. It entails being honest with each other, coming to decisions together, and making a commitment to your well-being. Together, you may create a personalized strategy for enhancing the health of your gut that might include dietary adjustments, prescription drugs, or other therapies.

Recall that improving your gut health is a journey, not a sprint. A mix of methods may be used, and medical specialists are essential in helping you achieve the best possible gut health. You're taking the initiative to live a better and more fulfilling life by identifying the warning signals that point to the need for expert assistance and selecting the best healthcare practitioner.

Long-Term Gut Health Maintenance

Greetings on your successful path to improved gut health! It's time to concentrate on sustaining and caring for your gut over the long term now that you have a thorough grasp of how your gut works, made healthy dietary and lifestyle adjustments and potentially sought advice from medical specialists. We'll look at the tactics and routines in this chapter that will support you in maintaining and improving your gut health over time.

1.Keep Things Consistent

Consistency is one of the cornerstones of gut health maintenance. Your everyday decisions shape the dynamic ecology that is your gut microbiota. Continue with the nutritional and behavioral adjustments you've made to make sure it thrives:

Diet: Keep up a varied, well-balanced diet high in fiber, probiotics, and prebiotics. Eating consistently contributes to the development of a stable and healthy gut microbiota.

Hydration: Keeping the gut healthy requires consuming enough water. Staying well-hydrated aids in the transportation of nutrients and aids in digestion.

Physical Activity: By encouraging a varied microbiota, regular exercise improves gut health. Strive for regular exercise to maintain the advantages.

Stress management: Stress has a detrimental effect on digestive health. Make time each day for stress-reduction exercises like yoga, meditation, or mindfulness.

Sleep: Give good sleep top priority. Your gut can heal and rebuild when you get regular, deep sleep, which has an impact on your physical and emotional health.

2.Continuous Self-Monitoring

It's simpler to keep up a gut-healthy lifestyle when you remain knowledgeable and conscious of your body's reactions. Take into account the following self-tracking techniques:

Food Diary: Keep recording your meals to track how your stomach reacts to various foods. Based on your findings, modify your diet as necessary.

Symptom Monitoring: Keep an eye out for any modifications to your digestive system. As soon as you become aware of recurrent symptoms, take action.

Frequent Check-Ins: To evaluate your gut health and get advice, make follow-up consultations with medical specialists regularly.

Lab Testing: Routine lab testing might provide information about the health of your intestines. Depending on what your healthcare professional recommends, these might include stool testing or other diagnostic procedures.

3.Remain Educated and Flexible

Research and learning about gut health are continuing. It's critical to keep updated since discoveries and ideas are always emerging:

Read and Learn: Stay up to date on the most recent findings around diet and gut health. Reputable websites, books, and articles may all be excellent sources of knowledge.

Speak with Experts: To modify your gut health plan, think about speaking with registered dietitians or medical specialists if your health changes or if new information becomes available.

4. Support and Community

Keeping your gut healthy may be a lifetime endeavour, and it can be more fun and sustainable if you have a supporting community:

Join Support Groups: If you have similar aspirations to others, you may want to consider joining support groups or communities. They may provide shared experiences, motivation, and support.

Tell Your Story: Tell your relatives and friends about your trip. Others may be motivated to emphasize gut health by your success.

Celebrate your accomplishments along the road as you make progress. To keep yourself motivated, celebrate your victories and accomplishments.

You may make sure that the improvements you've achieved are long-lasting by adopting these long-term gut health maintenance techniques into your everyday routine. You will be rewarded with increased vigor, well-being, and a lifetime of excellent health by your gut, which is a robust and flexible ecosystem. With a clear vision of a bright, healthy future, this chapter represents a fresh start when you take determined control of your path toward gut health.

Conclusion

Through our exploration of the complex realm of gut health in this book, we have come to realize that living a full and healthy life starts on the inside. There is no denying that there is a strong link between gut health and general well-being and that gut health is essential to our very lives.

We have looked at the microbiome, the vibrant community of bacteria living within us, and how they affect mood, immunity, digestion, and a host of other elements of our health. We now understand the critical role that nutrition plays, from the benefits of fiber and the symbiotic relationship between probiotics and prebiotics to the need to maintain enough hydration.

You now know how to create a diet that is both body and microbiota-nourishing and gut-healthy. You now have the resources to change your eating habits, from meal planning and nutritional selections to useful recipes.

However, our lifestyle choices have an impact on our gut health in addition to what we consume. We've looked at the significant effects of lifestyle decisions on our digestive systems, including the need to get enough sleep, manage stress, and exercise. Research on the mind-gut interaction has shown how closely our digestion and mental health are related.

As we come to the end of our trip, keep in mind that gut health is a lifetime commitment rather than a destination. It's about achieving balance, adopting healthy habits, and making well-informed decisions. In this lifetime endeavour, diagnosing and treating digestive health problems as well as working with medical experts when necessary are critical first steps.

You're investing in your future when you decide to give your gut health priority. You're welcoming a life full of vigour, resilience, and energy. You now have the power to nurture your gut, which is the key to realizing your greatest potential. I wish you well as you put this book down and start on your special road to a happier, healthier life. Whether you're just starting or have already made big adjustments, keep in mind that every decision you make counts. Your well-being is based on every meal, deep breath, and peaceful night's sleep.